LOSE WEIGHT FOR GOOD

LOSE WEIGHT FOR GOOD

All Natural 100 Year Old Remedy

NENAD TUBIC

To order additional copies of this book, contact:
Xlibris Corporation
1-888-795-4274
www.Xlibris.com
Orders@Xlibris.com
101783

TABLE OF CONTENTS

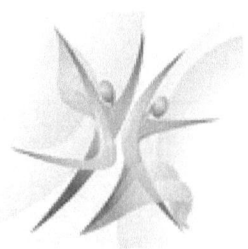

CHAPTER 1 –

INTRODUCTION

About a hundred years ago there were far fewer obese people than there are today. Believe it or not, only thirty years ago we were two times thinner.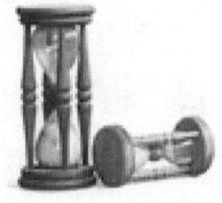

Today's lifestyle; the way we eat and the food quality, with all the chemical additives, as well as reduced physical activity are all contributing factors to today's obesity epidemic.

But in ancient times, people also ate fatty foods. At that time, there were no fitness centers or diet supplements for weight loss and yet, people were still thinner. Our grandmothers knew how to make natural and simple remedies to keep weight off. For example, people washed their hair without shampoo, which had not been invented, but their hair was more beautiful and healthier than ours today.

Diseases were cured only by natural means and these natural ways were the key to everything: good overall health, weight and spiritual life.

I received a few of these natural secrets from a nearly one hundred year old grandmother, who still remembers the remedies to staying slim. Even at that time people wanted to be slim and beautiful.

With her secrets, you can lose up to twenty pounds during the first month. Losing weight with this method is purely natural. Therefore, you will not feel dizzy, fatigued, or lose strength, common side effects to many diets. The solution includes normal daily food intake, without restriction. The body needs all the essential ingredients in order to function properly.

It is very important to know there is no diet, no mandatory exercise and no harmful pills, therefore there is no starvation, frustration or depression. There are only three secrets that are very simple, not time-consuming, and don't create an obligation or harmful habits. If you respect them, you will be forever slim. The greatest advantage to these three secrets is that the weight stays off, never comes back and there is no "yo-yo" effect.

Key facts according to data from the World Health Organization;[1]

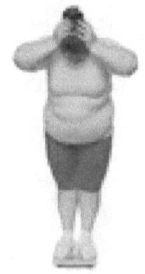

- Worldwide obesity has more than doubled since 1980.
- In 2008, 1.5 billion adults, 20 and older were overweight. Of these, over 200 million men and nearly 300 million women were obese.
- 65% of the world's population live in countries where obesity kills more people than being underweight.
- Nearly 43 million children under the age of five were overweight in 2010.
- Obesity is preventable.

Obesity occurs when caloric intake exceeds energy needs over a long period without energy expenditure. Then the excess calories are stored in the body in the form of energy reserves (glycogen and fat). These reserves are spent when needed, or if the body is starving.

Therefore, obesity will not occur if there is a balance between food intake and energy expenditure. Today, this

---

1   WWW.WHO.INT/ENTITY/MEDIACENTRE/FACTSHEETS/FS311/EN/

balance is almost impossible to maintain throughout life. But at the end of this e-book I will show you that it is possible in a very easy way without any dieting, exercise or harmful pills.

Many experts in obesity will tell you that diet and exercise are the first things you have to follow if you want to lose weight, but it's just not true. I want to be clear. All restrictive diets are very harmful. Losing weight in a short period does not mean the loss of fat from the body but the loss of water.

All exercise or any physical activity is very healthy for the overall state of the body and is a foundation for healthy living. It should certainly be performed as much as possible. This is not exclusively necessary in my weight loss method but if you do exercise, the effect will be quicker.

Obesity is defined as excess body fat. Obese people have more pounds than the ideal body weight, and the surplus is mostly fat (85%). The balance is a small part of water and muscle.

There are three levels of obesity; moderate obesity is the ideal body weight increased by 15%, distinct obesity is the ideal body weight increased by 25% and extreme obesity is the ideal body weight increased by more than 60%.

Women are more often obese. Obesity in women is most pronounced after twenty years of age and after menopause. Men often become overweight between 25 and 40 years of age.

We live in a time that is characterized by a rapid increase in obesity, due to modern lifestyles, which on the one hand means the consumption of energy-rich foods and on the other, reduced levels of physical activity.

Obesity has reached epidemic proportions. Particularly worrying is the fact that there is an increasing number 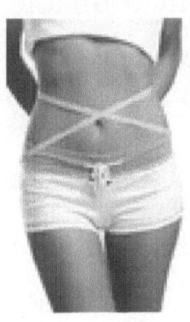 of obese children which usually grow into overweight adults. Obesity has the tendency to increase and become the leading public health issue. About 70% of men and women in the U.S. and about 50% in Europe are overweight and every fourth child.

To achieve the ideal body image, most women suffer. In a survey conducted in England, many of the respondents say they are ready to go to extreme steps to achieve the perfect look and weight. Approximately one third of the women surveyed said they would give at least one year of their life in exchange for slenderness.

The researchers note that although the data is quite shocking, it makes sense considering the global importance placed on women looking good. Currently feminine beauty is almost synonymous with slenderness. Pressures come from several different directions such as media, friends and family.

The survey also revealed that 46% of women said they were abused or ridiculed because of their looks. Looking good today is a preoccupation for many people.

In many countries around the world, the prevailing opinion is that managers and executives of large companies must not be obese. The explanation is if someone is unable to control their weight, they will not be able to control a company. Despite education, charm or skills, the candidate without weight problems will most often be selected. There are many other forms of discrimination tied to obesity that men and women face regularly. The assumption that obese people are bad workers is because they are inactive, slower to react and tire quickly, is used as an argument for favoring slender candidates. Physical beauty has become one of the main goals (or even "ideologies") of modern society. A body becomes a tool for achieving social promotion, strengthening professional or promoting personal status. Beauty, in other words, becomes usable, valuable "goods" for exchange and therefore, likely causes mass obsession with physical appearance.

CHAPTER 2 –

OBESITY AND HEALTH

Did you know that people with only ten percent more than their normal weight are exposed to increased risk of mortality by thirteen percent?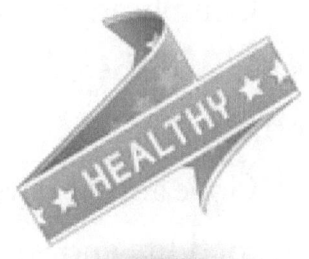

Today, a person generally begins the day with a coffee (and in many parts of the world, a cigarette), then goes to work, stopping at a shop along the way to pick up a quick snack if he gets hungry. He arrives home in the late afternoon, usually starving. He then proceeds to overeat, compensating for the day's lost meals. Stuffed, he lies on the couch in front of the TV. The four so-called "white death"; sugar, salt, white flour and fat, take their place on the main menu. He often only begins to worry about his health when he gets sick. Today, obesity has become more of a health problem than an aesthetic one.

Obesity is a serious chronic disease that can lead to many medical complications that reduce and shorten the quality of life, and whose treatments have a high price. Obese people are at risk of higher morbidity and mortality.

Each pound over the ideal body weight reduces life expectancy by one month.

Complications from obesity include a variety of diseases such as diabetes, arthritis, malignant diseases and many others.

Gone are the days when fatness was considered a symbol of good life and wealth.

A long time ago Hippocrates wrote: "Obesity is not just a disease, it is an indicator of other diseases." These other diseases include a number of complications from obesity.

The most known complication is metabolic syndrome, which results in a three times higher risk of stroke or heart attack. Obesity is a shortcut to diabetes. Adipose tissue has a dual role in the development of diabetes. High blood pressure is almost inevitable as a consequence of obesity. Many studies have shown that due to 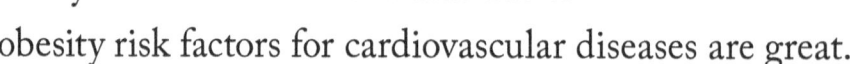 obesity risk factors for cardiovascular diseases are great.

It is less widely known that overweight people have a pulmonary function disorder, reduced total lung capacity and a very dangerous apnea (cessation of breathing for more than ten seconds), while sleeping. Nonalcoholic fatty liver is also a complication known to obesity. High cholesterol and symptomatic gallstones are six times more frequent than among slimmer people. Obesity damages joints, the spine, hips and knees sometimes to such an extent that movement is greatly impaired or impossible .

There is no doubt that obesity is a serious disease that reduces quality of life and longevity.

In addition to the physical health risks, mental health suffers from lack of enthusiasm, reduced self-esteem and confidence, depression, fewer chances for employment and relationships.

The food you eat can make you leaner or fatter which mostly depends on you. People prone to obesity have to be ready for radical changes.

CHAPTER 3 –

HEALTH COMES FIRST

Many people view a healthy lifestyle not only as something difficult to attain but unenjoyable. Traditional diets have taught us that if we want 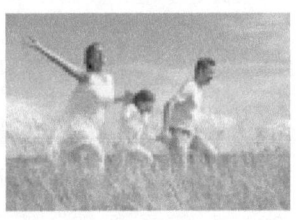 to lose weight, we have to count calories, keep track of everything we eat, and limit the amount and type of food we eat. Diets tell us exactly what and how much food to eat, not taking into account our preferences and individual relationships with hunger and satiety. Keeping to a diet in the short term can help you lose weight (fat, muscle and water), but it is so unnatural and so unrealistic that it can never become a lifestyle which we follow, let alone enjoy.

Most diets offer unrealistic recommendations and encourage health-threatening restrictions. More importantly, most diets do not teach us the safest, most effective ways of exercising, do not teach us how to deal with the desire for certain foods, or how to deal with the feelings of hunger and satiety. Sooner or later we will get bored of complexity, hunger, lack of taste, lack of flexibility, loss of energy and sense of deprivation.

The conclusion is quite logical; giving up the diet, returning to our starting weight and often, adding a few extra pounds.

Each time we start another diet, it becomes much more difficult to lose weight and we become more desperate and discouraged.

Then we begin to eat more and stick less to the diet, causing us more frustration, discouragement and depression. Soon, we find ourselves in a vicious circle. We begin to ask ourselves "Why bother?" We begin to blame ourselves for lack of strength and willpower. Deliberate restriction of food intake in order to lose weight or prevent weight gain, known as dieting, is the way that millions of people around the world try to live in order to keep up with society's coveted body image.

Preoccupation with body shape, size and weight creates an unhealthy lifestyle of emotional and physical restrictions. Diets deprive us of control over our lives. Many who diet lose the ability to eat in response to their physical needs. Weight loss by following a rigid diet is most often temporary. Most diets are too drastic to be regularly carried out, are unrealistic and unpleasant, physically and emotionally stressful and most of us just resume to our old habits related to diet and exercise.

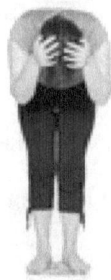

Diets control us, while we are not in control. Simply put, very few people are able to successfully implement a lifetime of dieting.

The reason why nearly all diets fail is very simple.

When we go on a low-calorie diet, our body thinks we are starving and it actually goes on the defensive and preserves fat by slowing down our metabolism. The moment we stop this way of eating or when we stop dieting, our metabolism continues to be slow and inefficient. We then gain weight even more rapidly, even though we might now be eating less than when we were on the diet. DIET

Low calorie diets also cause us to lose both muscle and fat in equal amounts. However, when we regain the weight, it's all fat, not muscle, resulting in an even slower metabolism. The end result is; heavier than before we started the diet, our body composition is less healthy and has a less attractive physique. This is called the yo-yo effect.

For example; if you normally consume 2500 calories per day, your body has adapted to this and burns 2500 calories a day. If you suddenly try starving yourself by consuming 1000 calories a day, your metabolism will adjust and only burn 1000 calories a day. That's why previous attempts at starvation fail. You must enter enough fat and protein to run your metabolism and maintain good health.

Diets ask us to sacrifice hunger. They do not allow us to enjoy the foods we like. Many diet programs force people to lower their caloric intake to dangerously low levels.

The common theory is that if you eat fewer calories than you burn, you will lose weight. This is true until such a time as you lower your caloric intake to a level that is lower than what your body needs to maintain essential life activities. This way you actually lose lean body mass, not fat. Your body dissolves its own muscle tissue to provide the needed energy to survive.

Your body is a machine that needs a certain amount of food at regular intervals throughout the day. If you do not eat certain foods at certain times, then the body will turn excess calories into fat. You should eat more than three times a day in order to lose weight.

If you skip breakfast in the morning, this will slow down your metabolism. If your largest meals are in the afternoon or evening, then the calories consumed are stored as fat. You should not have to starve or run marathons to lose weight.

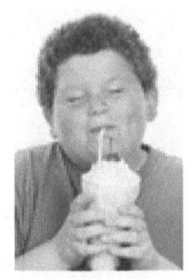

If you eat small portions or skip meals and yet it seems that everything sticks to you, this is not a coincidence. By skipping meals, you slow down your metabolism and it leads to a reduction in energy consumption. The reduced energy intake of valuable substances causes the body to save energy which is transformed into fat.

Fasting diets, which mostly attract those who want to lose weight, are the most dangerous to your health and should be avoided. It is important to know that weight loss due to fasting diets is actually the loss of liquids, not fat. So, pounds that disappear quickly will quickly return as soon as the liquid is compensated.

Health comes first and should not be questioned even at the cost of excess weight. Starvation is the most widespread method of removing the weight because it gives quick, but temporary results. Since it brings little or no calories, weight is lost, and the body feeds on itself. Nutrients taken from the muscle mass are as much as 50%.

This is a completely unacceptable way to lose weight and does not solve the problem of fat as it's muscle mass that is lost. People who are losing weight in this way appear unhealthy and exhausted.

The trend of thin and slender bodies seems to have reached a peak. Everybody wants to lose weight, and particularly in the summer time many people follow diets. The market is flooded with supplements that promise weight loss. But which ones really work?

CHAPTER 4 –

BIOLOGICAL FOOD VALUE

For a healthy and properly functioning body, you must 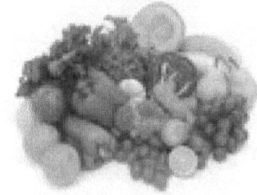 consume all the ingredients necessary for the renewal of cells in ideal quantities. Food builds, maintains and refreshes our body.

Organic food has a much greater biological value than food produced in a conventional manner; higher dry matter content, not artificially inflated with water and contains a higher percentage of vitamins and biologically active substances with significantly lower nitrate content (that cause cancer). These foods maintain freshness and composition longer. For 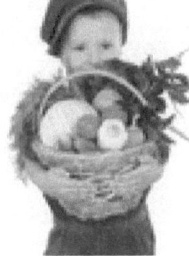 example, organically produced tomatoes contain 8-10% dry matter, while the chemical variety, 4-5%. Organic tomatoes stay fresh longer than a week in the refrigerator, while the chemical variety, only 2-3 days. Organic food has high nutritional and biological value, contains no harmful substances, gives the body strength, is fresher, and tastes better.

It is believed that fruit is the most valuable food consumed into the body, because it contains an ideal balance of the five essential elements that are essential for the body, which are glucose, amino acids, minerals, fatty acids and vitamins. When we talk about fruit, we refer only to fresh fruit because processed fruit loses much of its value.

Vegetables represent an important role in nutrition. Their nutritional value is assessed primarily by the content of minerals and vitamins. Vegetables are an even better source of vitamins than fruits. Some types of vegetable contain so much vitamin C, it's enough to take a dose of only 30-50 grams in order to meet the body's daily needs. For example, parsley leaves contain 166 mg% of vitamin C while fresh peppers contain 139 mg% of vitamin C. Vegetables contain other vitamins such as E, K, B1, B2, B6 and others.

Depending on the type of vegetable, the total amount of minerals range from 600–2200 mg in 100g of the edible part of the vegetable.

In fruit and all kinds of vegetables, potassium comprises the largest part of the overall total amount of mineral matter. Calcium, phosphorus and magnesium are also found in large quantities.

Proteins are essential to the diet to build and repair tissue, carbohydrates are for heat and energy, minerals are for bone structure, teeth, blood, etc., Vitamins are for promoting growth and preserving health and fiber is for the elimination of undigested matter.

Meat proteins are highly valuable because they contain a high proportion of essential amino acids. Meats contain all the amino acids necessary for good health.

There is one food group more important than all the others combined: water. Inadequate water intake gradually and imperceptibly can change the physiology of the organism and produces a range of chronic and degenerative changes to tissues and organs.

Believe it or not even diseases such as ulcers, high blood pressure, cholesterol, arthritis, allergies and asthma may be due to constant dehydration.

The above-mentioned facts are just a small sample of what's required for normal and healthy body function. Through restrictive diets, we do not consume many of the important substances listed above and this allows for possible complications in the body.

CHAPTER 5 –

IDEAL BODY WEIGHT

Ideal body weight is the weight that a person should have, taking into consideration a person's sex, age, longest life expectancy, maximum work capacity and optimum health.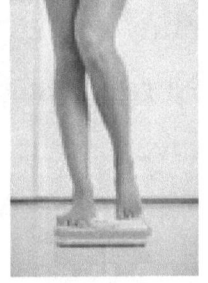

BMI (Body Mass Index) is the relationship between weight and height used to assess the impact of obesity as a risk factor to health. It is the mathematical formula that correlates with body fat in adults, and is calculated by weight (in kilograms) divided by body height (in meters squared).

For example, if you weigh 75 kilograms and are 1,74m tall, simply divide 75 by 1.74 m2. In this case, 24.8 is the BMI.

BMI	Nutritional status
< 18.5	Slim
>18.5 - 25	Normal weight
>25 – 30	Overweight
>30 – 35	Moderately obese
>35 – 40	Very obese
>40	Extremely obese

The BMI also can determine your health risk.

Nutritional status	Risk for the disease based on the BMI
Slim	Minimum
Normal weight	Low
Overweight	Moderate
Moderately obese	High
Very obese	Very high
Extremely obese	Extremely high

Ideal body weight can be calculated with formula as follows.

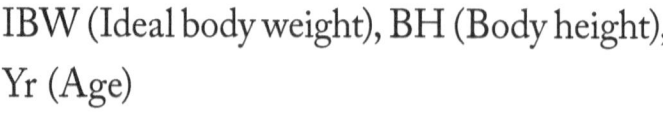

IBW (Ideal body weight), BH (Body height), Yr (Age)

For men: IBW = (BH-100) – (BH – 150/4) + (Yr – 20/4)

For women: IBW = (BH-100) – (BH-150/2.5) + (Yr – 20/4)

The simplest method of calculating ideal body weight is formula, where you subtract your height by 105 for women, or 100 for men to get the ideal body weight. This formula is not as reliable as the previous one.

The following table is a guide to a healthy weight range for each height and gender.

Height		Men		Women	
Feet & Inches	Metres	lb	Kg	lb	Kg
4' 7"	1.397	86 - 107	39 - 49	80 - 102	36 - 46
4' 7½"	1.410	88 - 109	40 - 49	82 - 104	37 - 47
4' 8"	1.422	90 - 111	41 - 50	83 - 106	38 - 48
4' 8½"	1.435	91 - 113	41 - 51	85 - 108	39 - 49
4' 9"	1.448	93 - 115	42 - 52	86 - 110	39 - 50
4' 9½"	1.461	95 - 117	43 - 53	88 - 112	40 - 51
4' 10"	1.473	96 - 119	44 - 54	89 - 114	41 - 52
4' 10½"	1.486	98 - 121	44 - 55	91 - 116	41 - 53
4' 11"	1.499	100 - 123	45 - 56	93 - 118	42 - 53
4' 11½"	1.511	101 - 125	46 - 57	94 - 120	43 - 54
5'	1.524	103 - 128	47 - 58	96 - 122	43 - 55
5' ½"	1.537	105 - 130	47 - 59	97 - 124	44 - 56
5' 1"	1.549	106 - 132	48 - 60	99 - 126	45 - 57
5' 1½"	1.562	108 - 134	49 - 61	101 - 128	46 - 58
5' 2"	1.575	110 - 136	50 - 62	102 - 130	46 - 59
5' 2½"	1.588	112 - 138	51 - 63	104 - 132	47 - 60
5' 3"	1.600	113 - 141	51 - 64	106 - 134	48 - 61
5' 3½"	1.613	115 - 143	52 - 65	107 - 137	49 - 62

Height		Men		Women	
Feet & Inches	Metres	lb	Kg	lb	Kg
5' 4"	1.626	117 - 145	53 - 66	109 - 139	49 - 63
5' 4½"	1.638	119 - 147	54 - 67	111 - 141	50 - 64
5' 5"	1.651	121 - 150	55 - 68	112 - 143	51 - 65
5' 5½"	1.664	123 - 152	56 - 69	114 - 145	52 - 66
5' 6"	1.676	125 - 154	56 - 70	116 - 147	53 - 67
5' 6½"	1.689	126 - 157	57 - 71	118 - 150	53 - 68
5' 7"	1.702	128 - 159	58 - 72	119 - 152	54 - 69
5' 7½"	1.715	130 - 161	59 - 73	121 - 154	55 - 70
5' 8"	1.727	132 - 164	60 - 74	123 - 157	56 - 71
5' 8½"	1.740	134 - 166	61 - 75	125 - 159	57 - 72
5' 9"	1.753	136 - 169	62 - 76	127 - 161	57 - 73
5' 9½"	1.765	138 - 171	63 - 78	128 -164	58 - 74
5' 10"	1.778	140 - 174	64 - 79	130 -166	59 - 75
5' 10½"	1.791	142 -176	64 - 80	132 - 168	60 - 76
5' 11"	1.803	144 - 179	65 - 81	134 - 171	61 - 77
5' 11½"	1.816	146 - 181	66 - 82	136 - 173	62 - 78
6' 0"	1.829	148 - 184	67 - 83	138 - 176	63 - 80
6' ½"	1.842	150 - 186	68 - 84	140 - 178	63 - 81
6' 1"	1.854	152 - 189	69 - 86	142 - 180	64 - 82
6' 1½"	1.867	154 - 191	70 - 87	144 - 183	65 - 83
6' 2"	1.880	157 - 194	71 - 88	146 - 185	66 - 84
6' 2½"	1.892	159 - 197	72 - 89	148 - 188	67 - 85
6' 3"	1.905	161 - 199	73 - 90	150 - 190	68 - 86
6' 3½"	1.918	163 - 202	74 - 92	152 - 193	69 - 88
6' 4"	1.930	165 - 205	75 - 93	154 - 196	70 - 89

CHAPTER 6 –

THE THREE EASY SECRETS

There are three easy secrets to losing weight slowly and very effectively, passed on from my grandmother. You can lose up to twenty pounds during the first month. Losing weight with 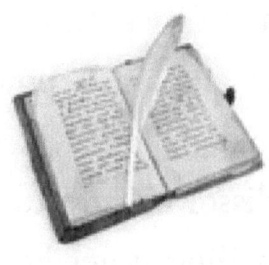 this method is purely natural. Therefore, you will not feel dizzy, fatigued, or lose strength, common side effects to many diets. The solution includes normal daily food intake, without restriction. The body needs all the essential ingredients in order to function normally.

It is very important to know there is no diet, no mandatory exercise, and no harmful pills therefore there is no starvation, frustration or depression. There are only three secrets that are very simple, not time–consuming, don't create an obligation or harmful habits. If you respect them, you will be FOREVER slim. The greatest advantage to these three secrets is that the weight STAYS OFF, NEVER comes back and there is NO "yo-yo" effect. Simple, easy and healthy? It is possible.

SECRET I

Every morning as soon as you wake up on an empty stomach about one hour before breakfast, as well as in the evening before bedtime drink this beverage prepared as follows: In one cup of boiling water, put ½ teaspoon of cinnamon powder. Wait until it becomes lukewarm and add one tablespoon of light colored honey. Mix until dissolved and drink slowly. Honey must not be put in boiling water because it loses its positive effects. When pouring the honey, DO NOT use a metal spoon. You may use a plastic, wooden, glass or ceramic tablespoon. Regularly consuming this beverage not only helps you lose weight but also prevents the accumulation of new fats.

If by any chance you are allergic to honey or cinnamon, do not consume this beverage. If you have a fever, do not consume cinnamon until the fever stops.

WHY HONEY AND CINNAMON

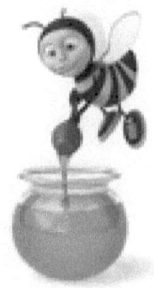

Though it may sound hard to believe, honey can help everyone with weight problems if you consume it the right way. You must be asking yourself how honey; high in calories, can actually help with weight loss. Honey is an all natural product with natural sugar.

Honey consists of a high percentage or fructose. The ratio between fructose and glucose is 1:1. Fruit has a similar ratio but it consists of much smaller quantities. Honey is much more favorable because you get the same results consuming smaller quantities.

Cinnamon slightly enhances body temperature to a level which we can't even feel, but one which is very important in the process of eliminating fatty substances. At the same time, honey feeds the adrenal gland so if we ingest just one spoon of honey in the evening, our metabolism works while we sleep at night.

In this way, we can actually live the fairytale of "losing weight while you sleep". The balanced intake of carbohydrates by honey reduces the hyperactivity of the adrenal gland and prevents the effects that their hormones trigger.

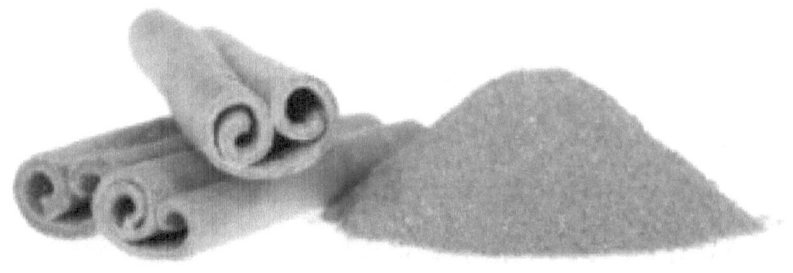

If those adrenal hormones are produced chronically, they lead to obesity and many other illnesses. Besides the good effects honey and cinnamon have on weight loss and the maintenance of body weight, they can heal a wide range of illnesses (used in different remedies) such as heart disease, arthritis, bladder infections, high cholesterol, hair loss, upset stomach, digestive problems, skin infection, etc.

SECRET 2

Before noon, drink the following tea: Put a tablespoon 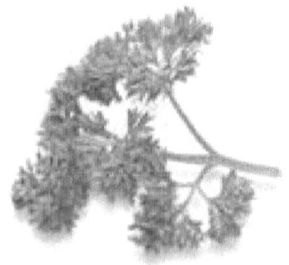 of dried parsley leaf tea and a pinch of parsley seeds (from fresh parsley flowers, not garden planting seeds) in a cup of cold water. Bring it to a boil, drain and drink while warm.

Do not drink it cold. If you cannot find parsley tea, you can dry it yourself.

Just take fresh parsley (leaves only) and spread them out on waxed paper in a dry and airy place, but not in the sun. It should be dried for the tea in two or three days. During the day, you may eat normal meals in moderate portions.

WHY PARSLEY TEA

Parsley is an aromatic plant which consists of a high level of vitamin C. In addition, parsley consists of high levels of apiol and miristicin and because of this, it is a very good diuretic and spasmolytic.

Because of the consistency of essential oils, parsley eliminates excess fluids in the stomach, leg and breast area. Parsley leaves are also effective against pain and inflammation. The most important benefit of parsley leaves in this case is that they function as a good diuretic, disposing of excess fatty substances through the urinal track.

SECRET 3

Supper has to be consumed before 7:00 p.m. It consists of homemade corn bread, made with corn flower (not polenta). Polenta is fattening.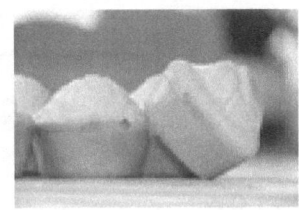

Alongside the bread, have a cup of unsweetened mint or chamomile tea or a cup of low fat yogurt.

HOMEMADE CORN BREAD:

2 eggs

½ cup oil

1 cup low fat sour cream

1 cup mineral water
  (room temperature)

2 cups corn flower

½ cup flower

1 teaspoon baking powder

Pinch of salt

150 grams cottage cheese
  (optional)

Preheat the oven at 220 degrees Celsius/440 degrees fahrenheit.

Beat eggs adding oil, sour cream, and mineral water. In a separate bowl, mix the flours together with the baking powder and salt then gradually add to the egg mixture. When well mixed, add the cottage cheese.

Pour the mixture into a muffin tin buttered and floured, do not use paper cups in the pan. Bake until golden for about 25 to 30 minutes. Great tasting corn bread made in less than 45 minutes.

Enjoy

NOTES

NOTES

Notes

Notes

NOTES

NOTES

Notes

NOTES

NOTES

NOTES

NOTES

Notes

www.ingramcontent.com/pod-product-compliance
Lightning Source LLC
Chambersburg PA
CBHW061227280526
45784CB00006B/2658